The Occupational Therapy Fieldwork

MANUAL FOR

ASSESSING

PROFESSIONAL

SKILLS

D1611769

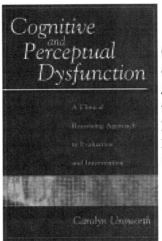
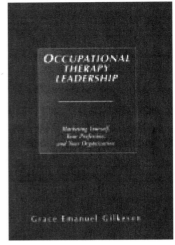
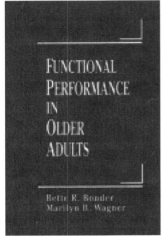
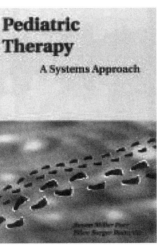

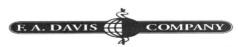

The Occupational Therapy Fieldwork MANUAL FOR ASSESSING PROFESSIONAL SKILLS

Judith Palladino, MA, OTR

Assistant Professor
Fieldwork Coordinator
Occupational Therapy Program
Department of Occupational Therapy
School of Allied Health Professions
Loma Linda University
Loma Linda, California

Ruth N. Jeffries, OTR

Fieldwork Coordinator
Extended Campus Coordinator
Occupational Therapy Assistant Program
Department of Occupational Therapy
School of Allied Health Professions
Loma Linda University
Loma Linda, California

 F. A. Davis Company • Philadelphia

F. A. Davis Company
1915 Arch Street
Philadelphia, PA 19103

Copyright © 2000 F. A. Davis Company

Printed in the United States of America

Last digit indicates print number: 10 9 8 7 6 5 4 3 2 1

Publisher: Jean-François Vilain
Senior Editor: Lynn Borders Caldwell
Production Editor: Jessica Howie Martin
Cover Designer: Louis J. Forgione

As new scientific information becomes available through basic and clinical research, recommended treatments and drug therapies undergo changes. The authors and publisher have done everything possible to make this book accurate, up to date, and in accord with accepted standards at the time of publication. The authors, editors, and publisher are not responsible for errors or omissions or for consequences from application of the book, and make no warranty, expressed or implied, in regard to the contents of the book. Any practice described in this book should be applied by the reader in accordance with professional standards of care used in regard to the unique circumstances that may apply in each situation. The reader is advised always to check product information (package inserts) for changes and new information regarding dose and contraindications before administering any drug. Caution is especially urged when using new or infrequently ordered drugs.

RM735
.P35
2000x
0 44124179

A NOTE TO THE EDUCATOR

The ability to take responsibility for one's own behavior is an important aspect in developing appropriate professional behaviors.[1]

Hughes & Opacich

WHY THIS BOOK IS NEEDED

The rapidly changing healthcare environment and heightened performance expectations have underscored the need to promote our students' professional socialization and professional identity. The incorporation of professional skill development into classroom and fieldwork settings must be a primary goal for healthcare educators. Developing effective professional behaviors empowers students to move with the healthcare system and adapt clinical skills to the demands or needs of a specific environment.[2]

Within the academic setting, professional skill development is frequently overlooked or not addressed until the latter portion of the student's fieldwork training. Established expectations and objectives for students in the Fieldwork Level I setting are sometimes minimal and inconsistently implemented by the fieldwork educator. For example, a student with above-average grades in course work may arrive late to class or a fieldwork assignment, answer a pager or cell phone during a treatment session, or respond defensively to feedback from the instructor or supervisor.

When professional skills are not assessed during academic and Fieldwork Level I experience, there is a greater potential for students to have difficulty in advanced levels of fieldwork because of inadequate professional socialization skills. Current literature, educator surveys, and interviews conducted by Loma Linda University faculty and students reveal that academic and fieldwork educators are experiencing increased frustration with their students' poor professional skills.

With valuable input from fieldwork educators, we developed this Fieldwork Level I manual to use as a professional skill assessment tool with our occupational therapy (OT) and occupational therapy assistant (OTA) students. At the request of fellow allied health professionals, we have made the manual more widely useable and applicable to a variety of disciplines and settings. Although the title, *The Occupational Therapy Fieldwork Manual for Assessing Professional Skills,* seems discipline specific, the practical approach of this manual allows it to be used by any health professional program.

HOW STUDENTS SHOULD USE THIS BOOK

The pages in this manual are three-hole punched and perforated so that students can put the pages in their own three-ring binders. Because the students take their manuals to each successive Fieldwork Level I assignment, each educator has an opportunity to review their past professional performance and the evaluative and technical skills attained. Having a student's progress recorded in one manual that is available to the student and educator can only strengthen the student's professional skills and foster communication among the student, academic educator, and fieldwork educator.

ADAPTING THE BOOK FOR YOUR FIELDWORK PROGRAMS

IN THE ACADEMIC SETTING

This manual can be adapted to the unique needs of individual fieldwork programs. Suggested options for its use include:

- Instructors can require satisfactory ratings on designated skill sheets for successful completion of their course.
- Instructors can require satisfactory performance on certain key behaviors on individual skill sheets for successful completion of their course.
- Instructors can require documentation on log sheets to reflect skill attainment and completion of course objectives.
- Satisfactory performance on identified key behaviors can be incorporated into a student professional portfolio that may be a requirement for graduation.

IN THE FIELDWORK SETTING

- Fieldwork educators can incorporate a review of the manual as part of the initial orientation with the student.
- Review of the fieldwork objectives and skill sheets can promote useful discussion and communication between student and supervisor regarding the student's strengths and weaknesses.
- In collaboration with the academic fieldwork coordinator, fieldwork educators can customize the fieldwork experience by designating certain key behaviors or individual skill sheets for assessment.
- In fieldwork sites where time for completion is a problem, educators can choose to complete only the one-page performance evaluation summary, using the skill sheets as a guide.

- Designated key behaviors can be used as a guide for developing learning and behavioral contracts with the student.
- Students can bring their manuals to their Fieldwork Level II affiliations to share their professional accomplishments and competencies attained in Fieldwork Level I. (The logs also give the fieldwork educator important information about the student's experience with evaluations, technical skills, and client exposure).

WHEN SEEKING EMPLOYMENT

Employers want to know that new graduates have demonstrated professional skills within their fieldwork assignments. Graduates can make the manual a component of their professional portfolio when seeking employment.

ACCREDITATION

All OT and OTA educational programs are required to document fieldwork experiences for accreditation. The table on pages viii–x demonstrates how this manual assists educational programs in meeting program and fieldwork accreditation standards for the Accreditation Council for Occupational Therapy Education (ACOTE) of the American Occupational Therapy Association, Inc.

FEEDBACK

We are very interested in hearing about your experiences with this manual. Please let us know how you use it and if you have any suggestions for its improvement. You can write to us at:

Judith Palladino and Ruth N. Jeffries
c/o Lynn Borders Caldwell
Senior Editor
F.A. Davis Company
1915 Arch Street
Philadelphia, PA 19103
Email: lbc@fadavis.com

REFERENCES

1. Hughes, C., and Opacich, K. (April, 1990). Academic Assessment Beyond the Cognitive Domain: Shaping Professional Behavior. Paper presented at Commission on Education, American Occupational Therapy Association Annual Meeting, New Orleans.

2. Crist, P. (1995). Students, it takes more than clinical skills to succeed. *Advance for Occupational Therapists, 11(16):5.*

ACOTE Standard For OTA Programs	ACOTE Standard For OT Programs	Skill Assessment Sheet No. in Manual
B 1.1 Demonstrate oral and written communication skills.	**B 1.1** Demonstrate oral and written communication skills.	5 – COMMUNICATION (General Skills) 6 – COMMUNICATION WITH STAFF 7 – COMMUNICATION WITH CLIENT 8 – WRITTEN COMMUNICATION
B 1.2 Employ logical thinking, critical analysis, problem-solving, and creativity.	**B 1.2** Employ logical thinking, critical analysis, problem-solving, and creativity.	1 – APPLICATION OF KNOWLEDGE/ CLINICAL REASONING 2 – COMMITMENT TO LEARNING
B 1.7 Demonstrate knowledge and appreciation of the role of sociocultural, socioeconomic, diversity factors, and lifestyle choices in contemporary society.	**B 1.7** Demonstrate knowledge and appreciation of the role of sociocultural, socioeconomic, diversity factors, and lifestyle choices in contemporary society.	7 – COMMUNICATION WITH CLIENT
B 1.8 Appreciate the influence of social conditions and the ethical context in which humans choose and engage in occupations.	**B 1.8** Appreciate the influence of social conditions and the ethical context in which humans choose and engage in occupations.	9 – PROFESSIONALISM
	B 3.6 Develop a basic understanding of theory development and its importance to occupational therapy.	1 – APPLICATION OF KNOWLEDGE/ CLINICAL REASONING
	B 4.4 Understand and appreciate the importance of cooperation with the occupational therapy assistant as a data gatherer and contributor to the screening and evaluation process.	10 – COOPERATION
B 3.3 Demonstrate the ability to use safety precautions with clients during the screening and evaluation process, such as standards for infection control that include, but are not limited to, universal precautions.	**B 4.8** Demonstrate the ability to use safety precautions with clients during the screening and evaluation process, such as standards for infection control that include, but are not limited to, universal precautions.	12 – SAFE BEHAVIOR IN THE FIELDWORK SETTING
B 4.2 Use individual and group interaction and therapeutic use of self as a means of achieving therapeutic goals.	**B 5.5** Use individual and group interaction and therapeutic use of self as a means of achieving therapeutic goals.	7 – COMMUNICATION WITH CLIENT 9 – PROFESSIONALISM

ACOTE Standard For OTA Programs	ACOTE Standard For OT Programs	Skill Assessment Sheet No. in Manual
B 4.6 Demonstrate the ability to interact through written, oral, and nonverbal communication with client/family/ significant others, colleagues, other health providers, and the public.	**B 5.9** Demonstrate the ability to interact through written, oral, and nonverbal communication with client/family/significant others, colleagues, other health providers, and the public.	5 – COMMUNICATION (General Skills) 6 – COMMUNICATION WITH STAFF 7 – COMMUNICATION WITH CLIENT 8 – WRITTEN COMMUNICATION
B 4.9 Demonstrate the ability to use safety precautions with the client during therapeutic intervention, such as contra-indications and use of infection control standards that include, but are not limited to, universal precautions.	**B 5.13** Demonstrate the ability to use safety precautions with the client during therapeutic intervention, such as contra-indications and use of infection control standards that include, but are not limited to, universal precautions.	12 – SAFE BEHAVIOR IN THE FIELDWORK SETTING
	B 5.14 Develop skills in supervising and collaborating with occupational therapy assistants on therapeutic interventions.	10 – COOPERATION
B 4.12 Monitor and reassess, in collaboraton with the client, the effect of occupational therapy interventions and the need for continued and/or modified intervention.	**B 5.16** Monitor and reassess, in collaboration with the client, the effect of occupational therapy interventions and the need for continued and/or modified intervention.	9 – PROFESSIONALISM
B 6.6 Use principles of time management, including being able to schedule and prioritize workloads.	**B 7.9** Use principles of time management, including being able to schedule and prioritize workloads.	3 – DEPENDABILITY/RESPONSIBILITY
B 7.3 Know when and how to find and use national and international informa-tional resources, including appropriate literature within and outside of occupa-tional therapy.	**B 8.3** Know when and how to find and use national and international informa-tional resources, including appropriate literature within and outside of occupational therapy.	4 – INITIATIVE
B 8.1 Demonstrate a knowledge and understanding of the AOTA Code of Ethics, Core Values and Attitudes of Occupational Therapy and AOTA Stand-ards of Practice as a Guide for profession-al interactions and in client treatment and employment settings.	**B 9.1** Demonstrate a knowledge and understanding of the AOTA Code of Ethics, Core Values and Attitudes of Occupation-al Therapy and AOTA Standards of Practice as a Guide for professional inter-actions and in client treatment and employ-ment settings.	9 – PROFESSIONALISM

continued

ACOTE Standard For OTA Programs	ACOTE Standard For OT Programs	Skill Assessment Sheet No. In Manual
B 8.6 Develop an understanding of personal and professional abilities and competencies as they relate to job responsibilities.	**B 9.6** Develop an understanding of personal and professional abilities and competencies as they relate to job responsibilities.	ENTIRE BOOK
B 8.8 Articulate the importance of professional relationships between the occupational therapist and the occupational therapy assistant.	**B 9.8** Articulate the importance of professional relationships between the occupational therapist and the occupational therapy assistant.	9 – PROFESSIONALISM 10 – COOPERATION
B 9.1 Document a plan to assure collaboration between academic and fieldwork representatives. The plan shall include agreed upon fieldwork objectives that are documented and made known to the student.	**B 10.1** Document a plan to assure collaboration between academic and fieldwork representatives. The plan shall include agreed upon fieldwork objectives that are documented and made known to the student.	ENTIRE BOOK
B 9.7 Document all Level I fieldwork experiences that are provided to students.	**B 10.7** Document all Level I fieldwork experiences that are provided to students.	ENTIRE BOOK
B 9.8 Document mechanisms for formal evaluations of student performance on Level I fieldwork.	**B 10.8** Document mechanisms for formal evaluations of student performance on Level I fieldwork.	ENTIRE BOOK

ACKNOWLEDGMENTS

We appreciate the time and effort that the following reviewers took to carefully read our manuscript and suggest improvements:

Marilyn L. Blaisdell, MA, OTR/L
Assistant Professor/Fieldwork Coordinator
Occupational Therapy Assistant Program
Becker College
Worcester, Massachusetts

Caryn Johnson, MS, OTR/L, FAOTA
Fieldwork Coordinator
Occupational Therapy Program
Thomas Jefferson University
Philadelphia, Pennsylvania

Nancy MacRae, MS, OTR/L, FAOTA
Associate Professor
Occupational Therapy Program
University of New England
Biddeford, Maine

Laura Lynn Swanson-Anderson, OTR/L
Fieldwork Coordinator
Occupational Therapy Program
St. Ambrose University
Davenport, Iowa

Marla Wonser, OTR/L
Program Director
Occupational Therapy Assistant Program
Casper College
Casper, Wyoming

CONTENTS

A NOTE TO THE EDUCATOR . . . . **v**
WHY THIS BOOK IS NEEDED   v
HOW STUDENTS SHOULD USE THIS BOOK   vi
ADAPTING THE BOOK FOR YOUR FIELDWORK PROGRAMS   vi
    In the Academic Setting   vi
    In the Fieldwork Setting   vi
    When Seeking Employment   vii
ACCREDITATION   vii
FEEDBACK   vii
REFERENCES   vii

HOW TO USE THIS MANUAL . . . . **xv**
GENERAL INSTRUCTIONS   xv
    1. Suggested Fieldwork Level I Objectives   xv
    2. Optional Fieldwork Level I Assignments   xvi
    3. Fieldwork Orientation Log   xvi
    4. Skill Assessment Sheets (Skills # 1–12)   xvi
    5. Fieldwork Educator Information   xvii
    6. Academic Educator Information   xviii
    7. Evaluation/Assessment Log   xviii
    8. Technical Skills Log   xviii
    9. Client Data Log   xix
    10. Performance Evaluations   xix
    11. Student Profile   xx
    12. Professional Documents   xx
    13. Miscellaneous Documentation and Resources   xx
DOCUMENTATION OF STUDENT PERFORMANCE   xxi
    General Guidelines   xxi
    Directions for the Student   xxi
    Directions for the academic and fieldwork educator   xxiii
    Directions for the academic fieldwork coordinator   xxiv
FINAL COMMENT   xxv
BIBLIOGRAPHY   xxv

1   **SUGGESTED FIELDWORK LEVEL I OBJECTIVES** **1**

2   **OPTIONAL FIELDWORK LEVEL I ASSIGNMENTS** **3**

③ **FIELDWORK ORIENTATION LOG** 5

④ **SKILL ASSESSMENT SHEETS** 7
SAMPLE OF A COMPLETED SKILL SHEET 8
SKILL #1: APPLICATION OF KNOWLEDGE/CLINICAL REASONING 9
SKILL #2: COMMITMENT TO LEARNING 11
SKILL #3: DEPENDABILITY/RESPONSIBILITY 13
SKILL #4: INITIATIVE 15
SKILL #5: COMMUNICATION (General Skills) 17
SKILL #6: COMMUNICATION WITH STAFF 19
SKILL #7: COMMUNICATION WITH CLIENT 21
SKILL #8: WRITTEN COMMUNICATION 23
SKILL #9: PROFESSIONALISM 25
SKILL #10: COOPERATION 27
SKILL #11: STRESS MANAGEMENT 29
SKILL #12: SAFE BEHAVIOR IN THE FIELDWORK SETTING 31

⑤ **FIELDWORK EDUCATOR INFORMATION** 33

⑥ **ACADEMIC EDUCATOR INFORMATION** 35

⑦ **EVALUATION/ASSESSMENT LOG** 39

⑧ **TECHNICAL SKILLS LOG** 43

⑨ **CLIENT DATA LOG** 47

⑩ **PERFORMANCE EVALUATIONS** 51
TIME SHEET 1 52
PERFORMANCE EVALUATION SUMMARY 1 53
TIME SHEET 2 54
PERFORMANCE EVALUATION SUMMARY 2 55
TIME SHEET 3 56
PERFORMANCE EVALUATION SUMMARY 3 57
TIME SHEET 4 58
PERFORMANCE EVALUATION SUMMARY 4 59

⑪ **STUDENT PROFILE** 61

⑫ **PROFESSIONAL DOCUMENTS** 63

⑬ **MISCELLANEOUS DOCUMENTATION AND RESOURCES** 65

HOW TO USE
THIS MANUAL

GENERAL INSTRUCTIONS

The pages in this manual are three-hole punched and perforated so that students can place them in a three-ring binder. Students may also want to purchase plastic tabs or tabbed dividers to make finding each section easier.

Listed below are the 13 major sections in this manual, along with their respective goals, descriptions, and directions for use.

The following terminology is used to describe the three different types of educators:

- Fieldwork educator: the mentor/instructor for the student at the fieldwork site
- Academic educator: the classroom instructor at an academic institution
- Academic fieldwork coordinator: the instructor at the academic institution who arranges the fieldwork locations for the students, acts as the liaison between the student and the fieldwork educators, and evaluates the students' fieldwork experience

1. SUGGESTED FIELDWORK LEVEL I OBJECTIVES

Goal

To aid in the development of general fieldwork objectives and guide the fieldwork experience.

Description

This is a list of suggested fieldwork objectives for both OT and OTA students that can apply to a variety of fieldwork settings.

How to Use

During the orientation meeting with the student, the fieldwork educator refers to these objectives and deletes, modifies, or adds to them to meet the needs of the program. Review of the objectives is included in the final evaluation progress.

2. OPTIONAL FIELDWORK LEVEL I ASSIGNMENTS

Goal

To aid in the development of fieldwork assignments.

Description

These are suggested, optional assignments that an OT or OTA program can use.

How to Use

The fieldwork educator reviews these assignments with the student, designates those that are required by the fieldwork program, and modifies them to meet the needs of the student and program.

3. FIELDWORK ORIENTATION LOG

Goal

To serve as a record of the student's fieldwork orientations.

Description

This log records the date and type of orientation and includes space for the coordinator's signature.

How to Use

The orientation log is an effective way to monitor the contacts between the student and the academic fieldwork coordinator. An initial orientation meeting with students should be scheduled at the beginning of the academic year to review the manual and explain its use. Subsequent meetings between the student and the academic fieldwork coordinator are recorded in this log.

4. SKILL ASSESSMENT SHEETS (SKILLS #1–12)

Goal

To provide an accurate picture of the student's professional behavior in designated skill areas. *On completion of the final fieldwork experience (before the initiation of Fieldwork Level II), each student is expected to have mastered a majority of **all** the key behaviors on every skill sheet.*

Description

There are 12 Skill Assessment Sheets (skill sheets), one sheet per skill area. Each sheet has a set of key behaviors, or performance criteria. There are four vertical columns to record key behavior ratings by the educator and by the student for each fieldwork experience and each designated academic class.

How to Use

The educator, using the Key Behavior Performance Rating Scale located on each sheet (sample on page xvii), rates the student on each key behavior.

KEY BEHAVIOR PERFORMANCE RATING SCALE

S+	Student has exceeded satisfactory performance Place an "S+" opposite the key behavior when the performance is above that expected of a student.
S	Student has performed at a satisfactory level Place an "S" opposite the key behavior when satisfactory performance is achieved and the behavior is consistent.
NE	Student needs experience Write "NE" opposite the key behavior if satisfactory performance has been demonstrated, but not at a consistent level. The student needs further experience. Please comment on what experience is needed.
NI	Student needs improvement Write "NI" opposite the key behavior if performance is inconsistent or requires supervision to be safe and effective. Comments describing why the performance needs improvement or is not yet independent are **required.**
N/O	Student has not had opportunity to work on key behavior Write "N/O" if there has been "no opportunity to perform" or this is not a skill that can be addressed in your setting.
—	Student was not evaluated on this key behavior Draw (—) if student was not evaluated on this key behavior during this fieldwork/classroom experience.

Students also rate their own performances using the same rating scale. Because fieldwork sites and classroom settings vary, students may not be evaluated on *all* the key behaviors on each skill sheet. In addition, they may not achieve a satisfactory level on each key behavior after just one or two fieldwork experiences.

5. FIELDWORK EDUCATOR INFORMATION

Goal

To serve as a record of the fieldwork educators who have evaluated/mentored the student.

Description

The fieldwork educator records his or her name and initials and the fieldwork site address in the order in which the student completes each fieldwork assignment.

How to Use

The Fieldwork Educator Information sheet provides an accurate, written record of each fieldwork experience. The academic fieldwork coordinator can refer to this record when he or she needs to contact an educator regarding the student's professional performance. Students also find this information useful when formulating a fieldwork experience or reference list during the employment process.

6. ACADEMIC EDUCATOR INFORMATION

Goal

To serve as a record of the academic educators who have evaluated/mentored the student.

Description

The academic educator records the class title and number and his or her name and initials.

How to Use

This information provides an accurate written record of each course instructor who evaluated the student's professional behavior. The academic work coordinator refers to this record when he or she needs to contact an instructor regarding the student's performance.

7. EVALUATION/ASSESSMENT LOG

Goal

To serve as a record of informal and formal interviews, evaluations, and assessments completed by the student in the classroom and fieldwork setting.

Description

Students are responsible for recording the date of administration, fieldwork or class number, type of evaluation/assessment, and level of independence (observed, with assistance, or independent). Students are also responsible for obtaining the initials of the academic and/or fieldwork educator for each entry.

How to Use

The assessments/evaluations vary from one fieldwork site to another and are based on each setting's needs. The log can aid academic and fieldwork educators in planning future classroom or fieldwork experiences and provides students with a complete record of their evaluation/assessment accomplishments.

8. TECHNICAL SKILLS LOG

Goal

To serve as a record of technical procedures, modalities, skills, and activities performed by the student in the classroom and fieldwork setting.

Description

Students are responsible for recording:

- Date performed
- Fieldwork or class number
- Specific type of technical skill
- Level of independence

Students are also responsible for obtaining the initials of the academic and/or fieldwork educator for each entry.

How to Use

The technical skills required may vary from one fieldwork site to another, based on each setting's needs. Review of this log will help academic and fieldwork educators plan future classroom or fieldwork experiences. The log also provides students with a complete record of technical skill accomplishments for future reference by the student.

9. CLIENT DATA LOG

Goal

To serve as a record of client diagnoses and performance deficits observed by the student in the classroom or fieldwork setting.

Description

Students are responsible for recording information on clients, including:

- Date observed
- Age and sex of client
- Client diagnosis
- Occupational performance areas and components affected
- Treatment interventions
- Equipment

How to Use

Review of this log will help academic and fieldwork educators plan future classroom or fieldwork experiences. It provides a useful, detailed record of client diagnoses seen and the treatment interventions applied for future reference by the student.

10. PERFORMANCE EVALUATIONS

Goal

To provide a summary of the student's professional performance on each fieldwork assignment and selected classroom settings.

Description

The Performance Evaluation includes:

- Time sheet (completed by the student)
- Summary form, which documents student performance and indicates successful or unsuccessful completion of the fieldwork assignment (completed by educator)
- Copy of each of the 12 individual Skill Assessment Sheets

How to Use

One performance evaluation must be completed for each Fieldwork Level I experience. The educator documents areas of strength and those needing improvement and reviews these with the student at the end of the fieldwork experience. The time sheet provides verification of hours spent in this fieldwork setting. The student should mail or deliver a copy of each Skill Assessment Sheet to the academic fieldwork coordinator. Originals should remain in the student's manual. These documents are part of the student's permanent departmental record.

11. STUDENT PROFILE

Goal

To provide information that may be useful in designing the optimal educational experience for the student.

Description

This section can include documents that profile the student's temperament, learning style(s), and other information that may help the educator to "know" the student better.

How to Use

These documents should be reviewed at the beginning of the fieldwork experience. The educator can then employ the teaching approaches and methods that are most appropriate for the student's learning style. Knowledge of the student's temperament will provide valuable insight into the student's responses to the fieldwork environment.

12. PROFESSIONAL DOCUMENTS

Goal

To collect important professional documents that the student can use during the educational program and keep for reference as a practitioner.

Description

These documents can include professional Code of Ethics, Standards of Practice, Uniform Terminology, or other similar professional resources.

How to Use

These documents are referred to and used by the student as needed in the classroom or fieldwork setting.

13. MISCELLANEOUS DOCUMENTATION AND RESOURCES

Goal

To provide a space for extra forms and other documents related to professional skill development.

Description

These documents and resources can include, but are not limited to, article reviews, task analyses, case studies, client interviews and assessments, and special assignments.

How to Use

These documents are additional information about and examples of the student's work in the classroom or fieldwork setting. They can provide important information about the student's writing ability and documentation style.

DOCUMENTATION OF STUDENT PERFORMANCE

GENERAL GUIDELINES

- All recording should be in *permanent ink.*
- Corrections should be lined out and changes initialed by the person who made the change. Correction fluid should not be used.

DIRECTIONS FOR THE STUDENT

Overall Responsibilities

You are responsible for:

- Completing the top portion of each of the 12 Skill Assessment Sheets
- Completing the information at the top of the Performance Evaluation Summary Form
- Recording the specified information in the logs
- Recording your self-ratings on the Skill Assessment Sheets
- Completing Time Sheets
- Mailing or delivering the Performance Evaluation to the academic fieldwork coordinator if requested to do so

You are expected to take primary responsibility for achieving acceptable mastery of a skill and take advantage of and seek opportunities that will facilitate mastery and promote learning. You are fully responsible for retaining and updating the manual.

Recording on the Skill Assessment Sheets

Rate your own performance during the course of the fieldwork. The fieldwork educator determines the timing of the self-assessment at the beginning of the fieldwork experience. Self-rating helps the educator determine how accurately you are assessing your own performance.

Classroom setting

- Rate your own performance in the space labeled *Student.*
- In the column corresponding to the fieldwork or academic course number, record the level of performance of *each* key behavior on the

individual skill assessment sheets, using the rating scale on page xvii for your assessment.

Fieldwork I setting

• Rate your own performance in the space labeled *Student*.

• In the column corresponding to the fieldwork or academic course number, record the level of performance for *each* key behavior on the individual skill assessment sheets, using the rating scale on page xvii for your assessment.

You will review and discuss these ratings with your fieldwork educator.

Recording on Logs

You are responsible for recording entries onto the log sheets as follows:

Evaluation/Assessment Log

• Date

• Fieldwork/class # (number)

• Type of evaluation or assessment

In this section, list the specific evaluations or assessments that you are exposed to by name, if applicable. For example, in occupational therapy, the assessments listed may include the Allen Cognitive Levels (ACL), Manual Muscle Test (MMT), and Peabody Developmental Motor Scales.

Your academic or fieldwork educator will initial each entry and check your performance level.

Technical Log

• Date

• Fieldwork/class # (number)

• Type of technical skill

In this section, list the specific technical skills to which you are exposed. For example, in occupational therapy, the list may include transfer training—bed to wheelchair, body mechanics, joint protection, work simplification, and group facilitation.

Your academic or fieldwork educator will initial each entry and check off your performance level.

Client Data Log

• Date

• Age

• Diagnosis

• Occupational Performance Areas Affected (Refer to Uniform Terminology for Occupational Therapy)

• Performance Components Affected (Refer to Uniform Terminology for Occupational Therapy)

• Treatment Interventions Observed

• Equipment Used

Time Sheet

Complete the Time Sheet, tabulate your total hours, and submit the sheet to your fieldwork educator for review and signature at the end of the fieldwork experience.

DIRECTIONS FOR THE ACADEMIC AND FIELDWORK EDUCATOR

Recording on the Skill Assessment Sheets

- Document your ratings in the space labeled *Educator*. Fieldwork settings are reserved for the first four columns; classroom settings are reserved for the second four columns.

- In the column corresponding to the appropriate fieldwork or academic course number, record the student's level of performance for *each* key behavior on the individual Skill Assessment Sheets, using the Key Behavior Performance Rating Scale that is printed on the reverse side of each skill sheet.

- You may rate a student at a higher or lower level of performance than at a previous fieldwork site or class, or your rating may concur with the previous evaluator. If the student is not evaluated on a key behavior, draw a horizontal line (—) in the box. For each fieldwork experience, all key behaviors should be rated by using one of the symbols described in the rating scale.

- If you give a student an *NE* (Student Needs Experience) rating, you may wish to add a comment. If you give a student an *NI* (Student Needs Improvement) rating, a comment is required. Record these remarks on your corresponding Performance Evaluation Summary. (See below for further details regarding the Performance Evaluation Summary.)

Fieldwork Educator/Academic Educator Information Forms

Fieldwork Educator

Record the Fieldwork Level I, your name, the fieldwork site name and address, and your initials.

Academic Educator

Record the class number, your name, the school name and address, and your initials.

Recording in Logs

You are responsible for:

- Initialing each student entry on the Evaluation/Assessment and Technical Skills Logs

- Checking off the level of student performance on the Evaluation/Assessment and Technical Skills Logs.

Performance Evaluation Forms

Fieldwork Educator

The Fieldwork Level I Performance Evaluation is a summary of the student's performance during each fieldwork experience. Complete one Performance

Evaluation at the end of the fieldwork experience. The complete evaluation for each site includes a:

- Time Sheet
- Performance Evaluation Summary
- Copy of each of the completed 12 Skill Assessment Sheets

The student will mail or deliver the Time Sheet and Performance Evaluation Summary to the academic educator. The Skill Assessment Sheets will remain in the student's manual and the student will hand-carry them to the fieldwork facility and school.

Time Sheet: Review and sign the time sheet after the student completes it.

Performance Evaluation Summary: Write specific comments here summarizing the student's performance, including those required when a student receives an *NI* rating.

Check *Yes* or *No* to indicate whether or not the student has successfully completed the Fieldwork I assignment. *Yes* means that the student will receive a *satisfactory grade* and does *not* require an additional fieldwork assignment in this practice area. *No* means that the student will receive an *unsatisfactory grade* and will need an additional fieldwork assignment in this practice area.

Both the *student* and *educator MUST SIGN the evaluation,* indicating review and discussion. The student will return all of these documents to the academic fieldwork coordinator by mail or in person. These documents are part of the student's permanent departmental record.

DIRECTIONS FOR THE ACADEMIC FIELDWORK COORDINATOR

After the student completes each fieldwork experience, you should:

- Review the Performance Evaluation
- Review the student's manual, including the skill sheets, logs, assignments, and documentation created during the fieldwork experience
- Assess skill mastery

Assessment of Skill Mastery

Review each skill sheet to determine the student's level of mastery to date. It may take several or all fieldwork experiences and/or classes to have all key behaviors rated at satisfactory or higher on each skill sheet. This review of skill mastery allows you to monitor student progress and intervene as necessary.

Complete the top box of each skill sheet as follows:

Skill Acceptance

Skill Acceptance is located in the table at the top of each skill sheet and occurs when *ALL of the key behaviors have received a satisfactory or higher rating.* Following your review of the student's manual, record the date, fieldwork number, and your initials under *Skill Acceptance.*

Skill Challenged

Skill Challenged occurs when a previously accepted skill is found to be deficient (below satisfactory) in one or more key behaviors at a subsequent fieldwork site or classroom (the educator has recorded an *NE* or *NI* in the corresponding key behavior column assigned to that Fieldwork Level I, or class). Following your review of the student's manual, record the date, fieldwork number, and your initials under *Skill Challenged,* indicating that the student's overall mastery of that skill area is below the satisfactory level on that particular fieldwork experience.

Skill Reaccepted

Skill Reaccepted occurs when deficiencies are eliminated and all performance levels are again at satisfactory or higher. Following your review of the student's manual, enter the date, fieldwork number, and your initials under *Skill Reaccepted.*

Final Evaluation

Once you have assessed the student's skill mastery and have reviewed the student's completed manual, share this information with the entire academic team and then meet with the student.

The final passing score for each Fieldwork Level I experience should be based on the Performance Evaluations, skill mastery achieved, faculty feedback, and supporting documentation. The performance expectation of each student should increase with each successive fieldwork experience.

FINAL COMMENT

As you go through the process of implementing and using this manual, please remember that it is a flexible document that can be customized to fit the needs of your particular academic program. We invite you to be as creative in its use as possible, and to promote it as a positive and useful tool for the student, fieldwork educators, and academic program.

BIBLIOGRAPHY

American Occupational Therapy Association, Inc. (1983). *AOTA Fieldwork Evaluation Form for Occupational Therapy Assistant Students.*

American Occupational Therapy Association, Inc. (1987). *AOTA Fieldwork Evaluation for the Occupational Therapist.*

Barnes, A., and Evenson, M. (April 1995). *Tufts University—BSOT; Level I Professional Development Monitor.* Paper presented at Commission on Education, American Occupational Therapy Association Annual Meeting, Denver, Colorado.

Bastian, M. (April 1995). *Facilitating Development of Professional Behaviors. Use of Generic Abilities Assessment.* Paper presented at Commission on Education, American Occupational Therapy Association Annual Meeting, Denver, Colorado.

Bator, L., Graves, S., Jacaban, D., Henson, J., Monahan, P., and Verdugo, P. (February 1996). *What are the Most Essential Health Skills Utilized by Registered Occupational Therapists and Where are They Acquired?* Paper presented at the Loma Linda University Senior Colloquium, Loma Linda, California.

Cohn, E., and Crist, P. (1995). Back to the future: New approaches to fieldwork education. *American Journal of Occupational Therapy* 49(2):156-159.

Foto, M. (1995). New President's Address: The future—Challenges, choices, and changes. *American Journal of Occupational Therapy 49(10):*955-959.

Herzberg, G. (1994). The successful fieldwork student: Supervision perceptions. *American Journal of Occupational Therapy 48(9):*817-823.

Kasar, J., and Watson, D. (April 1995). *Developing Professional Behaviors Across the Curriculum.* Paper presented at Commission on Education, American Occupational Therapy Association Annual Meeting, Denver, Colorado.

Kramer, P., and Stern, K. (1995). Approaches to improving student performance on fieldwork. *American Journal of Occupational Therapy 49(2):*156-159.

Meyers, S. (1995). Exploring the costs and benefits drivers of clinical education. *American Journal of Occupational Therapy 49(2):*107-111.

Rose, C., and Davis, K. (April 1995). *Curriculum Development to Enhance Professionalism.* Paper presented at Commission on Education, American Occupational Therapy Association Annual Meeting, Denver, Colorado.

Sands, M. (1995). Readying occupational therapy assistant students for Level II Fieldwork: Beyond academics to personal behaviors and attitudes. *American Journal of Occupational Therapy 49(2):*150-152.

Texas Consortium for Physical Therapy Clinical Education, Inc. (1995). *The Blue MACS (Mastery and Assessment of Clinical Skills).*

Zimmerman, S. (1995). Cooperative education: An alternative Level I fieldwork. *American Journal of Occupational Therapy 49(2):*153-155.

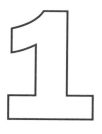

SUGGESTED FIELDWORK LEVEL I OBJECTIVES

By the end of the Fieldwork I assignment, the student will satisfactorily complete the following:

- Communicate effectively with staff, clients, families, and caregivers.
- Identify common characteristics seen in clients with specified diagnoses.
- Report clear, concise verbal and written observations of occupational therapy.
- When appropriate, identify where specific information is located in a medical chart per chart review and have an understanding of medical terms used.
- Identify therapeutic activities that promote function and facilitate client recovery.
- Understand the role of each member of the interdisciplinary team and their relationship to each other.
- Demonstrate an understanding of professional behavior skills (i.e., time management, punctuality, and dress code).
- Adhere to the institution's policies and procedures.
- Consider and demonstrate consistent safety with clients.
- Demonstrate an understanding of client rights.
- Demonstrate an understanding of confidentiality.
- Demonstrate an understanding of how self is used as a therapeutic tool.
- Understand his or her role in relationship to service delivery.
- Identify adaptive and assistive devices frequently used with the client.
- Be aware of the community resources available to the client and caregiver.
- Have an understanding of how a human being is an integration of many realms: physical, emotional, and social.

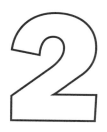

OPTIONAL FIELDWORK LEVEL I ASSIGNMENTS

These assignments are suggestions and are always at the discretion of the fieldwork educator.

- Present one case study, orally and in writing.
- Correctly complete a gross range-of-motion assessment.
- Complete a simple dressing assessment or activity (or other daily living skill-related activity).
- Correctly complete a functional muscle test.
- Co-lead two group activities with clients, reporting with a written Activity Analysis on one group.
- Conduct a semi-structured or structured interview.
- Complete a home barrier assessment of one client, if feasible or appropriate to the facility.
- Complete a task analysis of an appropriate treatment or activity specific to the client diagnosis.
- Devise one piece of adaptive equipment, diagnosis specific, to be left with the facility.

FIELDWORK ORIENTATION LOG

Directions to the Academic Fieldwork Educator: Note here when the student had his or her first fieldwork orientation and was instructed on how to use this manual. If you check the manual periodically, note those dates here too.

Date	Type of Orientation	Academic Fieldwork Coordinator Signature

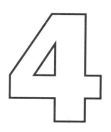

SKILL ASSESSMENT SHEETS

SAMPLE OF A COMPLETED SKILL SHEET

Student's Name: ___Jane Doe___

SKILL 1 Application of Knowledge / Clinical Reasoning		
Skill Acceptance	**Skill Challenged**	**Skill Re-accepted**
Date: 12-15-96	Date: 03-21-97	Date: 06-07-97
Fieldwork #: 2	Fieldwork #: 3	Fieldwork #: 4
AFC Initials: AZ	AFC Initials: NO	AFC Initials: RT

KEY BEHAVIORS		Fieldwork #				Class #				
		1	**2**	**3**	**4**	**OCTA 201**				
A Able to make pertinent and accurate observations.	**Student**	NE	NE	S	S					
	Educator	S	S	S+	S+	S				
B Raises relevant questions.	**Student**	NE	S	S	S+					
	Educator	S+	S+	S+	—	S+				
C Recognizes and identifies problems by using active listening and observation.	**Student**	NE	S	S+	S+					
	Educator	S	S	S	S+	S+				
D Gives alternative solutions to identified problems.	**Student**	NE	S	S	S					
	Educator	NE	S	S	S	S				
E Able to identify theory guiding practice (Frame of Reference).	**Student**	NI	NE	S	S+					
	Educator	S	S	S	S+	S+				
F Analyzes information. *Able to break down or separate basic information into parts.*	**Student**	S	S	S+	S+					
	Educator	S	S	S+	S+	S+				
G Synthesizes information. *Able to combine or integrate basic information.*	**Student**	NE	S	NE	S					
	Educator	NI	S	NE	S	S+				
H Interprets information. *Able to explain or clarify basic information.*	**Student**	S	S	S	S+					
	Educator	S	S	S	S+	S+				

S+ Exceeded Satisfactory Performance **S** Satisfactory Performance **NE** Needs Experience
NI Needs Improvement **N/O** No Opportunity **—** Not Evaluated

Student's Name: _____

SKILL 1 Application of Knowledge/Clinical Reasoning		
Skill Acceptance	**Skill Challenged**	**Skill Reaccepted**
Date:	Date:	Date:
Fieldwork #:	Fieldwork #:	Fieldwork #:
AFC Initials:	AFC Initials:	AFC Initials:

KEY BEHAVIORS		Fieldwork #				Class #			
		1	2	3	4				
A Able to make pertinent and accurate observations.	**Student**								
	Educator								
B Raises relevant questions.	**Student**								
	Educator								
C Recognizes and identifies problems by using active listening and observation.	**Student**								
	Educator								
D Gives alternative solutions to identified problems.	**Student**								
	Educator								
E Able to identify theory guiding practice (Frame of Reference)	**Student**								
	Educator								
F Analyzes information. *Able to break down or separate basic information into parts.*	**Student**								
	Educator								
G Synthesizes information. *Able to combine or integrate basic information.*	**Student**								
	Educator								
H Interprets information. *Able to explain or clarify basic information.*	**Student**								
	Educator								

S+ Exceeded Satisfactory Performance   **S** Satisfactory Performance   **NE** Needs Experience
NI Needs Improvement   **N/O** No Opportunity   — Not Evaluated

KEY BEHAVIOR PERFORMANCE RATING SCALE

S+   **Student has exceeded satisfactory performance**

Place an "S+" opposite the key behavior when the clinical performance is above that expected of a student.

S   **Student has performed at a satisfactory level**

Place an "S" opposite the key behavior when satisfactory performance is achieved and the behavior is consistent.

NE   **Student needs experience**

Write "NE" opposite the key behavior if satisfactory performance has been demonstrated, but not at a consistent level. The student needs further experience. Please comment on what experience is needed.

NI   **Student needs improvement**

Write "NI" opposite the key behavior if performance is inconsistent or requires supervision to be safe and effective. Comments describing why the performance needs improvement or is not yet independent are **required.**

N/O   **Student has not had opportunity to work on key behavior**

Write "N/O" if there has been "no opportunity to perform" or this is not a skill that can be addressed in your setting.

—   **Student was not evaluated on this key behavior**

Draw (—) if student was not evaluated on this key behavior during this fieldwork/classroom experience.

Student's Name: _____

SKILL 2 Commitment to Learning		
Skill Acceptance	**Skill Challenged**	**Skill Reaccepted**
Date:	Date:	Date:
Fieldwork #:	Fieldwork #:	Fieldwork #:
AFC Initials:	AFC Initials:	AFC Initials:

KEY BEHAVIORS		Fieldwork #				Class #				
		1	2	3	4					
A Identifies need for further information.	**Student**									
	Educator									
B Demonstrates positive attitude toward learning.	**Student**									
	Educator									
C Willingly accepts challenges and goes beyond minimum expectations.	**Student**									
	Educator									
D Puts new information into practice.	**Student**									
	Educator									
E Accepts the idea that there may be more than one answer to a problem.	**Student**									
	Educator									
F Offers own thoughts and ideas.	**Student**									
	Educator									
G Sets personal and professional goals.	**Student**									
	Educator									
H Actively seeks feedback.	**Student**									
	Educator									

S+ Exceeded Satisfactory Performance   **S** Satisfactory Performance   **NE** Needs Experience
NI Needs Improvement   **N/O** No Opportunity   — Not Evaluated

KEY BEHAVIOR PERFORMANCE RATING SCALE

S+   Student has exceeded satisfactory performance

Place an "S+" opposite the key behavior when the clinical performance is above that expected of a student.

S   Student has performed at a satisfactory level

Place an "S" opposite the key behavior when satisfactory performance is achieved and the behavior is consistent.

NE   Student needs experience

Write "NE" opposite the key behavior if satisfactory performance has been demonstrated, but not at a consistent level. The student needs further experience. Please comment on what experience is needed.

NI   Student needs improvement

Write "NI" opposite the key behavior if performance is inconsistent or requires supervision to be safe and effective. Comments describing why the performance needs improvement or is not yet independent are **required.**

N/O   Student has not had opportunity to work on key behavior

Write "N/O" if there has been "no opportunity to perform" or this is not a skill that can be addressed in your setting.

—   Student was not evaluated on this key behavior

Draw (—) if student was not evaluated on this key behavior during this fieldwork/classroom experience.

Student's Name: _____

SKILL 3 Dependability/Responsibility		
Skill Acceptance	**Skill Challenged**	**Skill Reaccepted**
Date:	Date:	Date:
Fieldwork #:	Fieldwork #:	Fieldwork #:
AFC Initials:	AFC Initials:	AFC Initials:

KEY BEHAVIORS		Fieldwork #				Class #				
		1	2	3	4					
A On time.	**Student**									
	Educator									
B Hands in assignments when due.	**Student**									
	Educator									
C Follows through with commitments and responsibilities.	**Student**									
	Educator									
D Respects others in the facility.	**Student**									
	Educator									
E Assumes responsibility for own actions.	**Student**									
	Educator									
F Uses time constructively in the fieldwork setting for learning opportunities.	**Student**									
	Educator									
G Prioritizes self and tasks.	**Student**									
	Educator									

S+ Exceeded Satisfactory Performance   **S** Satisfactory Performance   **NE** Needs Experience
NI Needs Improvement   **N/O** No Opportunity   — Not Evaluated

KEY BEHAVIOR PERFORMANCE RATING SCALE

S+   **Student has exceeded satisfactory performance**

Place an "S+" opposite the key behavior when the clinical performance is above that expected of a student.

S   **Student has performed at a satisfactory level**

Place an "S" opposite the key behavior when satisfactory performance is achieved and the behavior is consistent.

NE   **Student needs experience**

Write "NE" opposite the key behavior if satisfactory performance has been demonstrated, but not at a consistent level. The student needs further experience. Please comment on what experience is needed.

NI   **Student needs improvement**

Write "NI" opposite the key behavior if performance is inconsistent or requires supervision to be safe and effective. Comments describing why the performance needs improvement or is not yet independent are **required.**

N/O   **Student has not had opportunity to work on key behavior**

Write "N/O" if there has been "no opportunity to perform" or this is not a skill that can be addressed in your setting.

—   **Student was not evaluated on this key behavior**

Draw (—) if student was not evaluated on this key behavior during this field-work/classroom experience.

Student's Name: _____

SKILL 4 Initiative		
Skill Acceptance	**Skill Challenged**	**Skill Reaccepted**
Date	Date:	Date:
Fieldwork #:	Fieldwork #:	Fieldwork #:
AFC Initials:	AFC Initials:	AFC Initials:

KEY BEHAVIORS		Fieldwork #				Class #				
		1	2	3	4					
A Discusses related course assignments.	**Student**									
	Educator									
B Seeks and requests opportunities to gain new knowledge, e.g., literature, inservice programs.	**Student**									
	Educator									
C Makes use of own resources **before** asking for help.	**Student**									
	Educator									
D Self-starts own projects.	**Student**									
	Educator									
E Demonstrates assertiveness.	**Student**									
	Educator									

S+ Exceeded Satisfactory Performance   **S** Satisfactory Performance   **NE** Needs Experience
NI Needs Improvement   **N/O** No Opportunity   — Not Evaluated

KEY BEHAVIOR PERFORMANCE RATING SCALE

S+ Student has exceeded satisfactory performance

Place an "S+" opposite the key behavior when the clinical performance is above that expected of a student.

S Student has performed at a satisfactory level

Place an "S" opposite the key behavior when satisfactory performance is achieved and the behavior is consistent.

NE Student needs experience

Write "NE" opposite the key behavior if satisfactory performance has been demonstrated, but not at a consistent level. The student needs further experience. Please comment on what experience is needed.

NI Student needs improvement

Write "NI" opposite the key behavior if performance is inconsistent or requires supervision to be safe and effective. Comments describing why the performance needs improvement or is not yet independent are **required.**

N/O Student has not had opportunity to work on key behavior

Write "N/O" if there has been "no opportunity to perform" or this is not a skill that can be addressed in your setting.

— Student was not evaluated on this key behavior

Draw (—) if student was not evaluated on this key behavior during this fieldwork/classroom experience.

Student's Name: _____

SKILL 5 Communication (General Skills)		
Skill Acceptance	**Skill Challenged**	**Skill Reaccepted**
Date:	Date:	Date:
Fieldwork #:	Fieldwork #:	Fieldwork #:
AFC Initials:	AFC Initials:	AFC Initials:

KEY BEHAVIORS		Fieldwork #				Class #				
		1	2	3	4					
A Demonstrates active listening skills, e.g., eye contact, body language, verbal communication.	**Student**									
	Educator									
B Expresses information accurately, concisely, and clearly.	**Student**									
	Educator									
C Initiates communication in a timely manner.	**Student**									
	Educator									
D Adjusts verbal and nonverbal communication to each person and situation.	**Student**									
	Educator									
E Responds in a positive manner to questions, suggestions, and/or constructive criticism.	**Student**									
	Educator									

S+ Exceeded Satisfactory Performance   **S** Satisfactory Performance   **NE** Needs Experience
NI Needs Improvement   **N/O** No Opportunity   — Not Evaluated

KEY BEHAVIOR PERFORMANCE RATING SCALE

S+   Student has exceeded satisfactory performance

Place an "S+" opposite the key behavior when the clinical performance is above that expected of a student.

S   Student has performed at a satisfactory level

Place an "S" opposite the key behavior when satisfactory performance is achieved and the behavior is consistent.

NE   Student needs experience

Write "NE" opposite the key behavior if satisfactory performance has been demonstrated, but not at a consistent level. The student needs further experience. Please comment on what experience is needed.

NI   Student needs improvement

Write "NI" opposite the key behavior if performance is inconsistent or requires supervision to be safe and effective. Comments describing why the performance needs improvement or is not yet independent are **required.**

N/O   Student has not had opportunity to work on key behavior

Write "N/O" if there has been "no opportunity to perform" or this is not a skill that can be addressed in your setting.

—   Student was not evaluated on this key behavior

Draw (—) if student was not evaluated on this key behavior during this fieldwork/classroom experience.

Student's Name: _____

SKILL 6 Communication with Staff		
Skill Acceptance	**Skill Challenged**	**Skill Reaccepted**
Date:	Date:	Date:
Fieldwork #:	Fieldwork #:	Fieldwork #:
AFC Initials:	AFC Initials:	AFC Initials:

KEY BEHAVIORS		Fieldwork #				Class #			
		1	2	3	4				
A Polite, able to judge when to add input.	**Student**								
	Educator								
B Contributes in meetings when appropriate.	**Student**								
	Educator								
C Respects time limitations of others by being prepared for discussions and conferences.	**Student**								
	Educator								
D Able to share concerns and feelings regarding fieldwork experience with supervisor.	**Student**								
	Educator								

S+ Exceeded Satisfactory Performance **S** Satisfactory Performance **NE** Needs Experience
NI Needs Improvement **N/O** No Opportunity — Not Evaluated

KEY BEHAVIOR PERFORMANCE RATING SCALE

S+ Student has exceeded satisfactory performance

Place an "S+" opposite the key behavior when the clinical performance is above that expected of a student.

S Student has performed at a satisfactory level

Place an "S" opposite the key behavior when satisfactory performance is achieved and the behavior is consistent.

NE Student needs experience

Write "NE" opposite the key behavior if satisfactory performance has been demonstrated, but not at a consistent level. The student needs further experience. Please comment on what experience is needed.

NI Student needs improvement

Write "NI" opposite the key behavior if performance is inconsistent or requires supervision to be safe and effective. Comments describing why the performance needs improvement or is not yet independent are **required.**

N/O Student has not had opportunity to work on key behavior

Write "N/O" if there has been "no opportunity to perform" or this is not a skill that can be addressed in your setting.

— Student was not evaluated on this key behavior

Draw (—) if student was not evaluated on this key behavior during this fieldwork/classroom experience.

Student's Name: _____

SKILL 7 Communication with Client		
Skill Acceptance	**Skill Challenged**	**Skill Reaccepted**
Date:	Date:	Date:
Fieldwork #:	Fieldwork #:	Fieldwork #:
AFC Initials:	AFC Initials:	AFC Initials:

KEY BEHAVIORS		Fieldwork #				Class #				
		1	2	3	4					
A Nonjudgmental, culturally sensitive.	**Student**									
	Educator									
B Interacts with client-centered focus and demonstrates ability to establish rapport.	**Student**									
	Educator									
C Considers impact of interaction(s), both verbal and nonverbal, on client and/or caregiver.	**Student**									
	Educator									
D Uses appropriate body postures and gestures that suggest attentiveness, approachability, and acceptance.	**Student**									
	Educator									

S+ Exceeded Satisfactory Performance   **S** Satisfactory Performance   **NE** Needs Experience
NI Needs Improvement   **N/O** No Opportunity   — Not Evaluated

KEY BEHAVIOR PERFORMANCE RATING SCALE

S+   Student has exceeded satisfactory performance

Place an "S+" opposite the key behavior when the clinical performance is above that expected of a student.

S   Student has performed at a satisfactory level

Place an "S" opposite the key behavior when satisfactory performance is achieved and the behavior is consistent.

NE   Student needs experience

Write "NE" opposite the key behavior if satisfactory performance has been demonstrated, but not at a consistent level. The student needs further experience. Please comment on what experience is needed.

NI   Student needs improvement

Write "NI" opposite the key behavior if performance is inconsistent or requires supervision to be safe and effective. Comments describing why the performance needs improvement or is not yet independent are **required.**

N/O   Student has not had opportunity to work on key behavior

Write "N/O" if there has been "no opportunity to perform" or this is not a skill that can be addressed in your setting.

—   Student was not evaluated on this key behavior

Draw (—) if student was not evaluated on this key behavior during this fieldwork/classroom experience.

Student's Name: _____

SKILL 8 Written Communication		
Skill Acceptance	**Skill Challenged**	**Skill Reaccepted**
Date:	Date:	Date:
Fieldwork #:	Fieldwork #:	Fieldwork #:
AFC Initials:	AFC Initials:	AFC Initials:

KEY BEHAVIORS		Fieldwork #				Class #				
		1	2	3	4					
A Writes legibly; uses acceptable grammar and correct punctuation and spelling.	**Student**									
	Educator									
B Uses appropriate terminology and abbreviations approved by the facility.	**Student**									
	Educator									
C Communicates information accurately, clearly, and concisely in writing.	**Student**									
	Educator									

S+ Exceeded Satisfactory Performance   **S** Satisfactory Performance   **NE** Needs Experience
NI Needs Improvement   **N/O** No Opportunity   — Not Evaluated

KEY BEHAVIOR PERFORMANCE RATING SCALE

S+   Student has exceeded satisfactory performance

Place an "S+" opposite the key behavior when the clinical performance is above that expected of a student.

S   Student has performed at a satisfactory level

Place an "S" opposite the key behavior when satisfactory performance is achieved and the behavior is consistent.

NE   Student needs experience

Write "NE" opposite the key behavior if satisfactory performance has been demonstrated, but not at a consistent level. The student needs further experience. Please comment on what experience is needed.

NI   Student needs improvement

Write "NI" opposite the key behavior if performance is inconsistent or requires supervision to be safe and effective. Comments describing why the performance needs improvement or is not yet independent are **required.**

N/O   Student has not had opportunity to work on key behavior

Write "N/O" if there has been "no opportunity to perform" or this is not a skill that can be addressed in your setting.

—   Student was not evaluated on this key behavior

Draw (—) if student was not evaluated on this key behavior during this fieldwork/classroom experience.

Student's Name: _____

SKILL 9 Professionalism		
Skill Acceptance	**Skill Challenged**	**Skill Reaccepted**
Date:	Date:	Date:
Fieldwork #:	Fieldwork #:	Fieldwork #:
AFC Initials:	AFC Initials:	AFC Initials:

KEY BEHAVIORS		Fieldwork #				Class #				
		1	2	3	4					
A Abides by professional code of ethics.	**Student**									
	Educator									
B Abides by facility policy and procedures, e.g., dress code, schedule, use of phone, beeper, and so forth.	**Student**									
	Educator									
C Suitably dressed for environment and related tasks and activities.	**Student**									
	Educator									
D Conducts all client care activities with respect for the client's rights, e.g., confidentiality, modesty.	**Student**									
	Educator									
E Respects the right of those in authority to make decisions and complies with those decisions.	**Student**									
	Educator									
F Manages personal affairs in a manner that does not interfere with professional responsibilities.	**Student**									
	Educator									
G Modifies and maintains professional behavior according to demands of situation.	**Student**									
	Educator									

S+ Exceeded Satisfactory Performance   **S** Satisfactory Performance   **NE** Needs Experience
NI Needs Improvement   **N/O** No Opportunity   — Not Evaluated

KEY BEHAVIOR PERFORMANCE RATING SCALE

S+   Student has exceeded satisfactory performance

Place an "S+" opposite the key behavior when the clinical performance is above that expected of a student.

S   Student has performed at a satisfactory level

Place an "S" opposite the key behavior when satisfactory performance is achieved and the behavior is consistent.

NE   Student needs experience

Write "NE" opposite the key behavior if satisfactory performance has been demonstrated, but not at a consistent level. The student needs further experience. Please comment on what experience is needed.

NI   Student needs improvement

Write "NI" opposite the key behavior if performance is inconsistent or requires supervision to be safe and effective. Comments describing why the performance needs improvement or is not yet independent are **required.**

N/O   Student has not had opportunity to work on key behavior

Write "N/O" if there has been "no opportunity to perform" or this is not a skill that can be addressed in your setting.

—   Student was not evaluated on this key behavior

Draw (—) if student was not evaluated on this key behavior during this field-work/classroom experience.

Student's Name: _____

SKILL 10 Cooperation		
Skill Acceptance	**Skill Challenged**	**Skill Reaccepted**
Date:	Date:	Date:
Fieldwork #:	Fieldwork #:	Fieldwork #:
AFC Initials:	AFC Initials:	AFC Initials:

KEY BEHAVIORS		Fieldwork #				Class #				
		1	2	3	4					
A Works effectively with other individuals.	**Student**									
	Educator									
B Shows consideration for the needs of the group.	**Student**									
	Educator									

S+ Exceeded Satisfactory Performance   **S** Satisfactory Performance   **NE** Needs Experience
NI Needs Improvement   **N/O** No Opportunity   — Not Evaluated

KEY BEHAVIOR PERFORMANCE RATING SCALE

S+ Student has exceeded satisfactory performance

Place an "S+" opposite the key behavior when the clinical performance is above that expected of a student.

S Student has performed at a satisfactory level

Place an "S" opposite the key behavior when satisfactory performance is achieved and the behavior is consistent.

NE Student needs experience

Write "NE" opposite the key behavior if satisfactory performance has been demonstrated, but not at a consistent level. The student needs further experience. Please comment on what experience is needed.

NI Student needs improvement

Write "NI" opposite the key behavior if performance is inconsistent or requires supervision to be safe and effective. Comments describing why the performance needs improvement or is not yet independent are **required.**

N/O Student has not had opportunity to work on key behavior

Write "N/O" if there has been "no opportunity to perform" or this is not a skill that can be addressed in your setting.

— Student was not evaluated on this key behavior

Draw (—) if student was not evaluated on this key behavior during this fieldwork/classroom experience.

Student's Name: _____

SKILL 11 Stress Management		
Skill Acceptance	**Skill Challenged**	**Skill Reaccepted**
Date:	Date:	Date:
Fieldwork #:	Fieldwork #:	Fieldwork #:
AFC Initials:	AFC Initials:	AFC Initials:

KEY BEHAVIORS		Fieldwork #				Class #			
		1	2	3	4				
A Recognizes and manages own stress or problems by demonstrating effective coping skills.	**Student**								
	Educator								
B Recognizes stress or problems in others.	**Student**								
	Educator								

S+ Exceeded Satisfactory Performance   **S** Satisfactory Performance   **NE** Needs Experience
NI Needs Improvement   **N/O** No Opportunity   — Not Evaluated

KEY BEHAVIOR PERFORMANCE RATING SCALE

S+   Student has exceeded satisfactory performance

Place an "S+" opposite the key behavior when the clinical performance is above that expected of a student.

S   Student has performed at a satisfactory level

Place an "S" opposite the key behavior when satisfactory performance is achieved and the behavior is consistent.

NE   Student needs experience

Write "NE" opposite the key behavior if satisfactory performance has been demonstrated, but not at a consistent level. The student needs further experience. Please comment on what experience is needed.

NI   Student needs improvement

Write "NI" opposite the key behavior if performance is inconsistent or requires supervision to be safe and effective. Comments describing why the performance needs improvement or is not yet independent are **required.**

N/O   Student has not had opportunity to work on key behavior

Write "N/O" if there has been "no opportunity to perform" or this is not a skill that can be addressed in your setting.

—   Student was not evaluated on this key behavior

Draw (—) if student was not evaluated on this key behavior during this field-work/classroom experience.

Student's Name: _____

SKILL 12 Safe Behavior in the Fieldwork Setting		
Skill Acceptance	**Skill Challenged**	**Skill Reaccepted**
Date:	Date:	Date:
Fieldwork #:	Fieldwork #:	Fieldwork #:
AFC Initials:	AFC Initials:	AFC Initials:

KEY BEHAVIORS		Fieldwork #				Class #				
		1	2	3	4					
A Demonstrates awareness and use of Universal Precautions.	**Student**									
	Educator									
B Provides a safe environment to prevent injury.	**Student**									
	Educator									
C Asks for assistance when unable to handle clients independently.	**Student**									
	Educator									
D Uses proper guarding techniques, e.g., accurate body placement to protect client.	**Student**									
	Educator									
E Uses proper body mechanics when handling clients independently.	**Student**									
	Educator									
F Demonstrates safe handling of clients and equipment.	**Student**									
	Educator									
G Provides appropriate level of supervision for clients.	**Student**									
	Educator									
H Demonstrates awareness of the safety of other clients and persons in the immediate area.	**Student**									
	Educator									

S+ Exceeded Satisfactory Performance **S** Satisfactory Performance **NE** Needs Experience
NI Needs Improvement **N/O** No Opportunity — Not Evaluated

Educator: Please complete the Performance Evaluation.

KEY BEHAVIOR PERFORMANCE RATING SCALE

S+ Student has exceeded satisfactory performance

Place an "S+" opposite the key behavior when the clinical performance is above that expected of a student.

S Student has performed at a satisfactory level

Place an "S" opposite the key behavior when satisfactory performance is achieved and the behavior is consistent.

NE Student needs experience

Write "NE" opposite the key behavior if satisfactory performance has been demonstrated, but not at a consistent level. The student needs further experience. Please comment on what experience is needed.

NI Student needs improvement

Write "NI" opposite the key behavior if performance is inconsistent or requires supervision to be safe and effective. Comments describing why the performance needs improvement or is not yet independent are **required.**

N/O Student has not had opportunity to work on key behavior

Write "N/O" if there has been "no opportunity to perform" or this is not a skill that can be addressed in your setting.

— Student was not evaluated on this key behavior

Draw (—) if student was not evaluated on this key behavior during this field-work/classroom experience.

FIELDWORK EDUCATOR INFORMATION

Fieldwork #	Name of Fieldwork Educator & Address of Fieldwork Site (Please print clearly)	Initials

ACADEMIC EDUCATOR INFORMATION

Class Title/#	Name of Academic Educator (Please print clearly)	Initials

Class Title/#	Name of Academic Educator (Please print clearly)	Initials

Class Title/#	Name of Academic Educator (Please print clearly)	Initials

7

EVALUATION/ ASSESSMENT LOG

Directions to the student: Record each client evaluation and assessment that you have done in the classroom and fieldwork setting here. Have the educator check the appropriate box to indicate whether each evaluation/assessment was observed, performed with assistance, or performed independently. Ask your academic or fieldwork educator to initial each entry.

Date	Fieldwork #/ Class #	Educator's Initials	Type of Evaluation/ Assessment (Please indicate name of test if applicable)	Observed	With Assistance	Independent

Date	Fieldwork #/ Class #	Educator's Initials	Type of Evaluation/ Assessment (Please indicate name of test if applicable)	Observed	With Assistance	Independent

Date	Fieldwork #/ Class #	Educator's Initials	Type of Evaluation/ Assessment (Please indicate name of test if applicable)	Observed	With Assistance	Independent

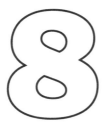

TECHNICAL SKILLS LOG

Directions to the Student: Use this log to record technical procedures, modalities, and skills that you have performed in both the classroom and fieldwork settings. Have the educator check the appropriate box to indicate whether each technical skill was observed, performed with assistance, or performed independently. Ask your academic or fieldwork educator to initial each entry.

Date	Fieldwork #/ Class #	Educator's Initials	Type of Technical Skill	Observed	With Assistance	Independent

Date	Fieldwork #/ Class #	Educator's Initials	Type of Technical Skill	Observed	With Assistance	Independent

Date	Fieldwork #/ Class #	Educator's Initials	Type of Technical Skill	Observed	With Assistance	Independent

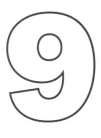

CLIENT DATA LOG

Directions to the student: Record client diagnoses, performance deficits, and interventions that you have observed in the classroom or fieldwork setting.

Date	Age	Sex	Diagnosis	Occupational Performance Areas Affected	Performance Components Affected	Treatment Interventions Observed	Equipment Used

Date	Age	Sex	Diagnosis	Occupational Performance Areas Affected	Performance Components Affected	Treatment Interventions Observed	Equipment Used

Date	Age	Sex	Diagnosis	Occupational Performance Areas Affected	Performance Components Affected	Treatment Interventions Observed	Equipment Used

10

PERFORMANCE EVALUATIONS

This section includes four copies of the time sheets and performance evaluation summaries so that one can be used for each of four fieldwork experiences.

TIME SHEET 1

Student: _____

Facility: _____

Time Period: _____

Directions to the Student: Complete the time schedule below for each Level I
Fieldwork experience.

Date	In	Out	In	Out	Hours	Comments

Total Hours _____

Fieldwork Educator Signature _____

PERFORMANCE EVALUATION SUMMARY 1

Student's Name: _____

Fieldwork #:_____   Quarter/Semester: _____   Year: _____

Facility: _____

Educator: _____

Summary/Comments (If the student received any "NI" [Needs Improvement] marks, please indicate why):

The student has successfully completed the fieldwork assignment and will receive a satisfactory grade.

☐   YES, the student does not need an additional fieldwork assignment in this practice area.

☐   NO, the student needs an additional fieldwork assignment in this practice area.

Please sign here to indicate review and discussion of this evaluation:

_____   _____
Signature (Fieldwork Educator)   Date   Signature (Student)   Date

Due by:

Return to:

TIME SHEET 2

Student: _____

Facility: _____

Time Period: _____

Directions to the Student: Complete the time schedule below for each Level I Fieldwork experience.

Date	In	Out	In	Out	Hours	Comments

Total Hours _____

Fieldwork Educator Signature _____

PERFORMANCE EVALUATION SUMMARY 2

Student's Name: _____

Fieldwork #: _____   Quarter/Semester: _____ Year: _____

Facility: _____

Educator: _____

Summary/Comments (If the student received any "NI" [Needs Improvement] marks, please indicate why):

The student has successfully completed the fieldwork assignment and will receive a satisfactory grade.

☐ YES, the student does not need an additional fieldwork assignment in this practice area.

☐ NO, the student needs an additional fieldwork assignment in this practice area.

Please sign to indicate review and discussion of this evaluation:

_____   _____
Signature (Fieldwork Educator)   Date   Signature (Student)   Date

Due by:

Return to:

TIME SHEET 3

Student: _____

Facility: _____

Time Period: _____

Directions to the Student: Complete the time schedule below for each Level I Fieldwork experience.

Date	In	Out	In	Out	Hours	Comments

Total Hours _____

Fieldwork Educator Signature _____

PERFORMANCE EVALUATION SUMMARY 3

Student's Name: _____

Fieldwork #:_____   Quarter/Semester: _____ Year: _____

Facility: _____

Educator: _____

Summary/Comments (If the student received any "NI" [Needs Improvement] marks, please indicate why):

The student has successfully completed the fieldwork assignment and will receive a satisfactory grade.

☐ YES, the student does not need an additional fieldwork assignment in this practice area.

☐ NO, the student needs an additional fieldwork assignment in this practice area.

Please sign to indicate review and discussion of this evaluation:

_____   _____
Signature (Fieldwork Educator)   Date   Signature (Student)   Date

Due by:

Return to:

TIME SHEET 4

Student: _____

Facility: _____

Time Period: _____

Directions to the Student: Complete the time schedule below for each Level I Fieldwork experience.

Date	In	Out	In	Out	Hours	Comments

Total Hours _____

Fieldwork Educator Signature _____

PERFORMANCE EVALUATION SUMMARY 4

Student's Name: _____

Fieldwork #:_____   Quarter/Semester: _____ Year: _____

Facility: _____

Educator: _____

Summary/Comments (If the student received any "NI" [Needs Improvement] marks, please indicate why):

The student has successfully completed the fieldwork assignment and will receive a satisfactory grade.

    ☐   YES, the student does not need an additional fieldwork assignment in this practice area.

    ☐   NO, the student needs an additional fieldwork assignment in this practice area.

Please sign to indicate review and discussion of this evaluation:

_____   _____

Signature (Fieldwork Educator)   Date   Signature (Student)   Date

Due by:

Return to:

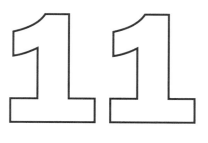

STUDENT PROFILE

Directions to the student: Place documents here that profile your learning style(s), temperament, and additional related information.

12

PROFESSIONAL DOCUMENTS

Directions to the student: Place professional documents here so that you can refer to them easily in the classroom or fieldwork setting. These documents may include your professional code of ethics, standards of practice, and uniform terminology.

13

MISCELLANEOUS DOCUMENTATION AND RESOURCES

Directions to the student: Place documents here that relate to professional skill development.